# Pain

# No More

## Fast & Easy Self Healing

## Methods

### By

### Alex Taurus

Alex Taurus

*This maybe isn't the first but is the last book you will ever need on healing...*

Alex Taurus

# **NOTICE**

The exercises published in this book do not replace medical recommendations in any way.

Not all exercises are suitable for you. In case of any doubts about any of the exercises contained herein, please consult your doctor.

If the exercise is accompanied by severe pain or discomfort, the exercise should be ended immediately and you should consult with your doctor.

Alex Taurus

# CONTENTS

Alex Taurus

# INTRODUCTION BY THE AUTHOR

Do you suffer from back pain after a long day at work? Do you suffer from leg pain after a long period of time on your feet? Do you suffer from neck pain from countless hours sitting at the computer?

**How do we solve these problems? The simplest solution is to seek a specialist.**

Unfortunately, nowadays, when we suffer from a complete lack of time, a visit to the specialist is often postponed until a time when the pain becomes unmanageable.

**A little about me**

I have been helping patients to eliminate their many different pains and aches over the last 28 years as a masseur and manual physiotherapist, and I created a methodology for the prevention and treatment of muscle pain, summarized in this book.

The book consists of the most effective and simple techniques and exercises that I recommend to my patients to accelerate healing at home and to prevent future disease.

This book is written in a simple and clear language with minimal use of expert medical terminology. The book targets a general audience primarily, and does not require medical qualifications, although I hope that experts will find a lot of useful information contained herein.

The aim of this book is to teach you how to eliminate muscular pain in a fast and effective manner.

To do so, it is required to learn these two simple principles:

1. Firstly, to remove the tension in the area of pain through **massage**.

2. Then, learn a suitable way to **stretch the muscles** in the area.

The stretching exercises focus on particular parts of the human body. Therefore, if you have problems in a specific area, you do not have to do all of the exercises in this book. In this case, I recommend after treatment of the painful area, if possible, to stretch all other surrounding areas as well.

For example, if you suffer from shoulder pain, I recommend a stretching of the neck muscles, cervical spine and arm after the stretching of the shoulder muscles.

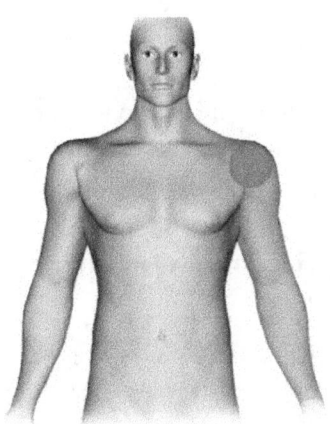

I would like to point out that this book is not a panacea. You should consult a medical specialist in case of serious pain. This book nevertheless teaches you how to treat the problem before reaching a critical point where the solution will be difficult even for medical experts.

# CHAPTER 1. PAINFUL POINTS

**What are the pain points?**

The center of each painful location is one or several points that extend the pain throughout the painful area.

**What do the painful points look like?**

These points are thickened points inside the muscles. They may feel firm, round and obviously painful to the human touch :-)

Massaging of these painful points is a simple, fast and effective method to eliminating muscle pain, which is more effective than the conventional limbering up of the muscles.

In general, we can eliminate or significantly reduce pain almost anywhere on the body through this simple method.

**How does it work?**

The human body is a body with a recuperative power controlled by the brain.

Massage of painful points is mainly in cooperation with the brain.

Acting on the painful point, we send a signal to the brain about the problem. The brain requires a lot of time to "accept" this signal and to "instruct" the correction of the problem. Therefore, in treating painful areas on your body, perform the following:

a) Sit down in a position in which the painful area is relaxed. The examples of such positions are given below.

b) Gradually palpate (feel) the painful zone and press on the most painful point with finger.

c) Press this point immediately until you feel an acceptable pain (for sending a signal to the brain).

**Attention**! The pain is a result of your touch, which sends a signal to the brain, but if you press a point too intensive and the pain increases, then the brain can send an "instruction" and instead of relaxing the bottleneck, it results in muscle spasm.

d) Press it within 10 to 30 seconds with the same pressure (do not increase or decrease a pressure) and allow some time for "the signal to be processed" by a brain.

**Attention**! Do not perform a traditional massage on this point, for example - circular movement. It affects and changes feelings, leading to disturbances (changes) of the "signal" transmitted to the brain. The brain does not understand what it can do.

Focus your attention on the ends of your fingers (close your eyes) and you feel that at this point the pain is melting away slowly and soon disappears or decreases greatly.

## 5. How to apply pressure to the pain points

You can press on a painful point with one finger.

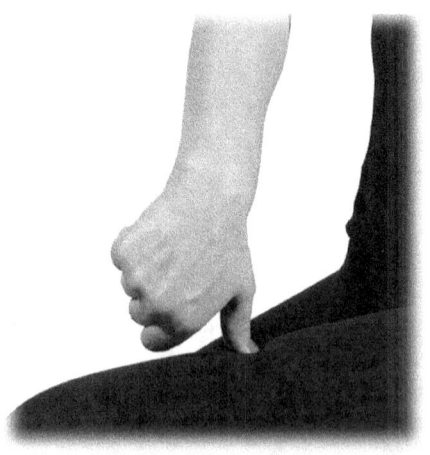

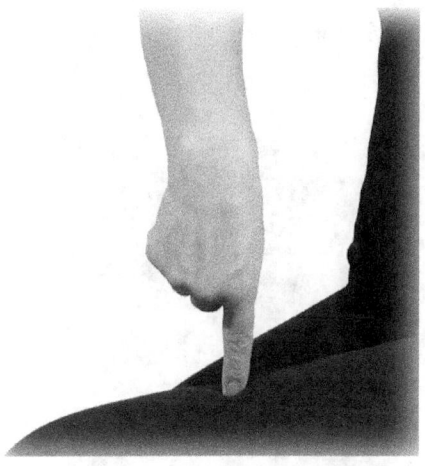

Or with a few fingers.

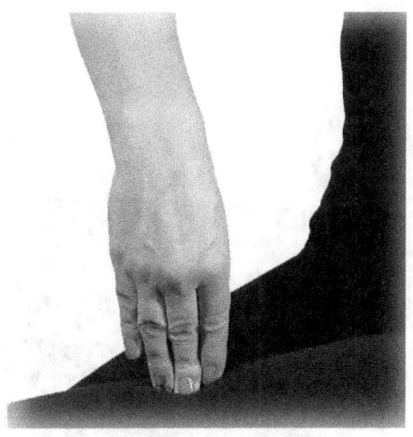

There are places where the painful point "disappears" (or jumps) beneath the touch of your fingers. In this case, you can press on painful point with your fingers so that you take muscle with fingers from both sides.

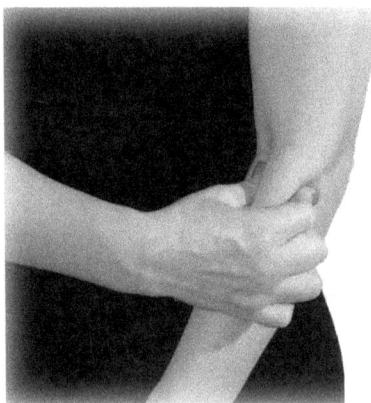

If you do not have a force strong enough to apply pressure, try to use your other hand if possible, or even your knuckle.

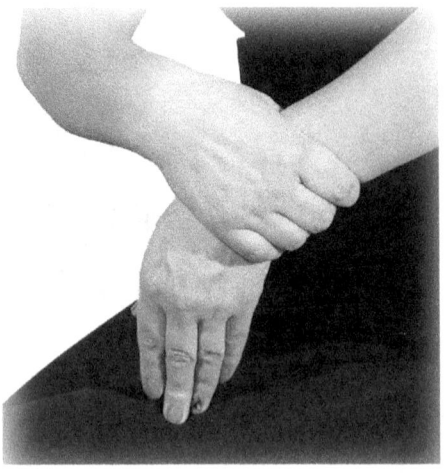

## 6. Learn to treat painful points

How it is done:

a) Sit down in a position where the painful area is relaxed,

b) Find the painful point,

c) Press this point until you feel an acceptable amount of pain,

d) Press the point for the next 10 to 30 seconds with the same force, until the pain disappears.

If there is more than one painful point in the same painful area of your body, firstly, treat the point that is most painful, then go to the next point. Perform the same procedure to treat all the points in that painful area.

The painful points on the head, the neck, the cervical spine, the chest and the abdomen, and hands and feet can be treated most simply because they are easily reachable by the hand. When treating a painful point in the neck, the cervical spine and the hands, it is more comfortable to sit on a table.

To relax the muscles of the cervical spine, lean on your elbows.

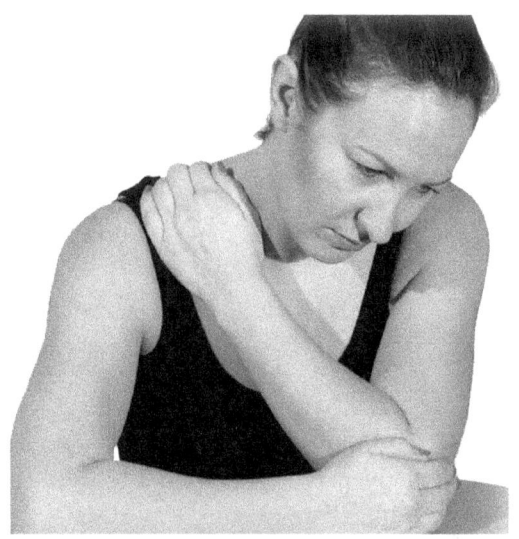

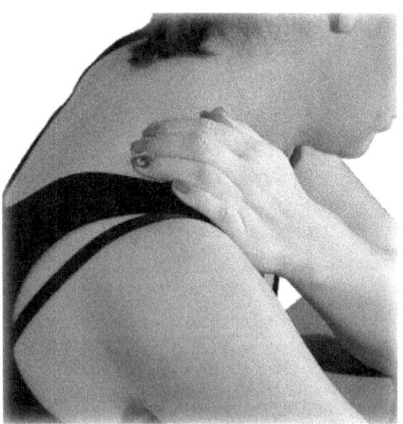

**Attention**! Seek and treat the points placed deep under the trapezoid muscle, between the clavicle and the first rib. Usually most of the problems arise with the cervical spine, although this area generally receives the least attention.

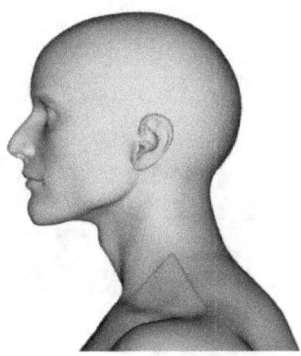

To relax the neck muscles, lean your forehead on one hand and treat the painful points with your other hand.

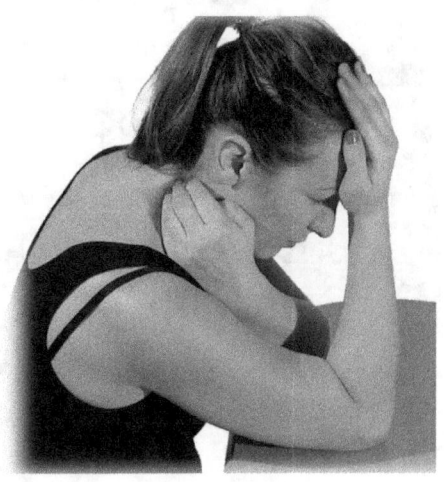

To relax the muscles of the hands, put one hand on the table and treat the painful point of the first hand by your second.

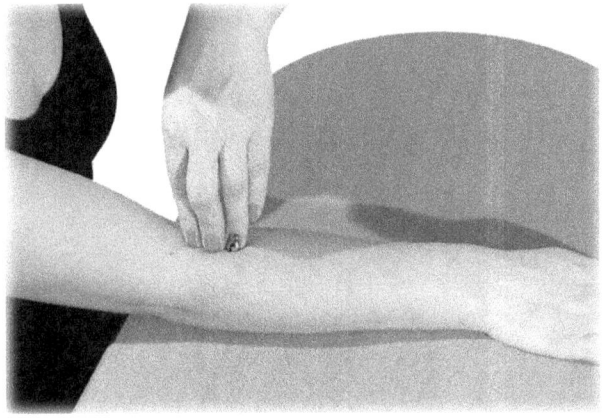

To treat foot pain, it is better to do it in a seated position because with this position you can use your other hand.

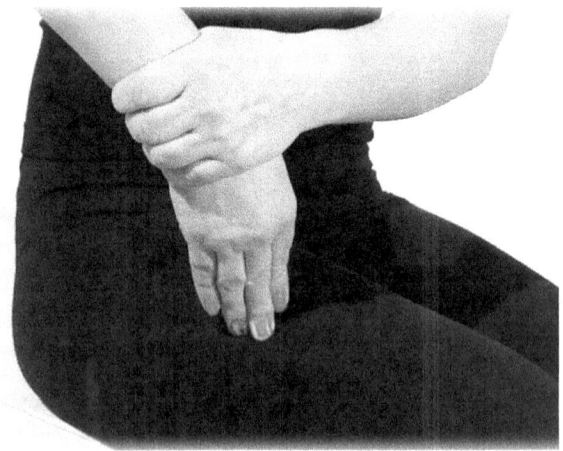

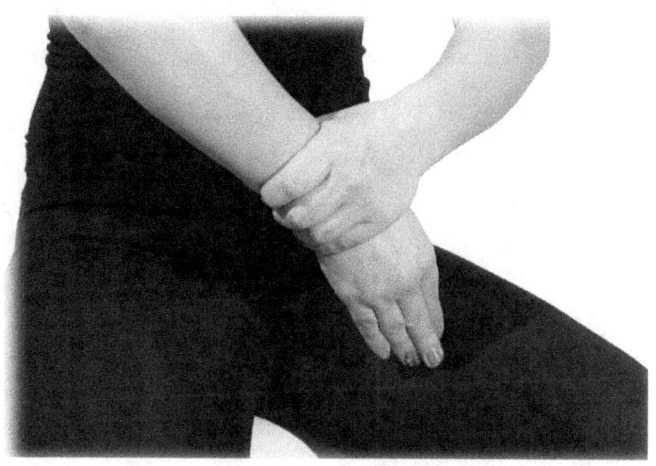

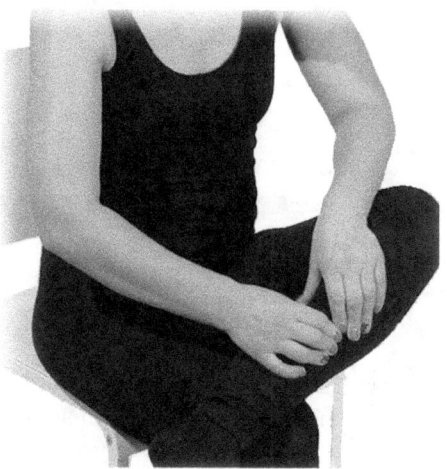

In most cases, you cannot reach pain points on the back by hand. In some cases, you can reach it, but it is difficult to press it or you do not have enough power. In this case, use ordinary available items such as furniture, i.e. unleash your imagination and use anything you can think of. The purpose is to find an object, which can press on a painful point and select a position in which you can also relax simultaneously.

**For example:**

You can lie down on your back and lean the painful point on the hardball (golf), chestnut, round stone, lid from a shampoo, etc. Choose the diameter of such object according to your feeling. The pain must be acceptable and you must be fully relaxed.

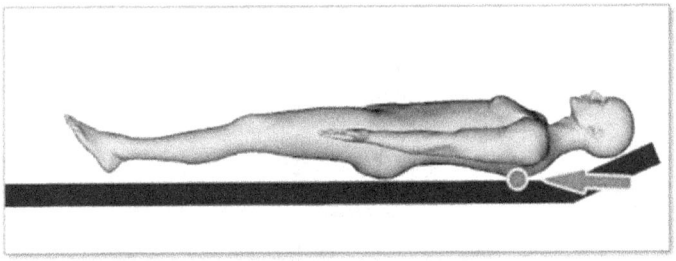

- You can lean on your back on the corner of the table, a cabinet or the holder in the tram.

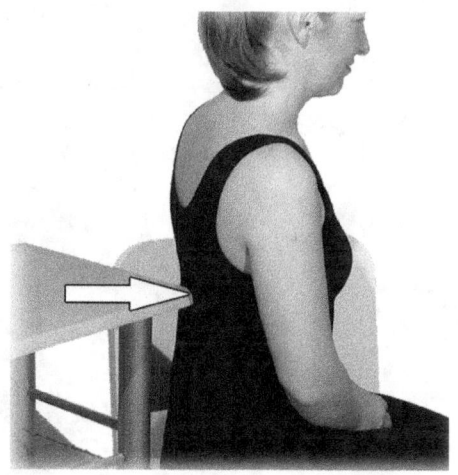

- You can use such subject with the rounded end to press on the points in the lumbar spine. For example, a broom with its one end leaning against a wall. It is recommended to lean such objects on something that is at the level of the lumbar spine, such on the (komod) chest or as the backrest of the chair. For a deeper massaging effect, you can treat the painful points from different angles.

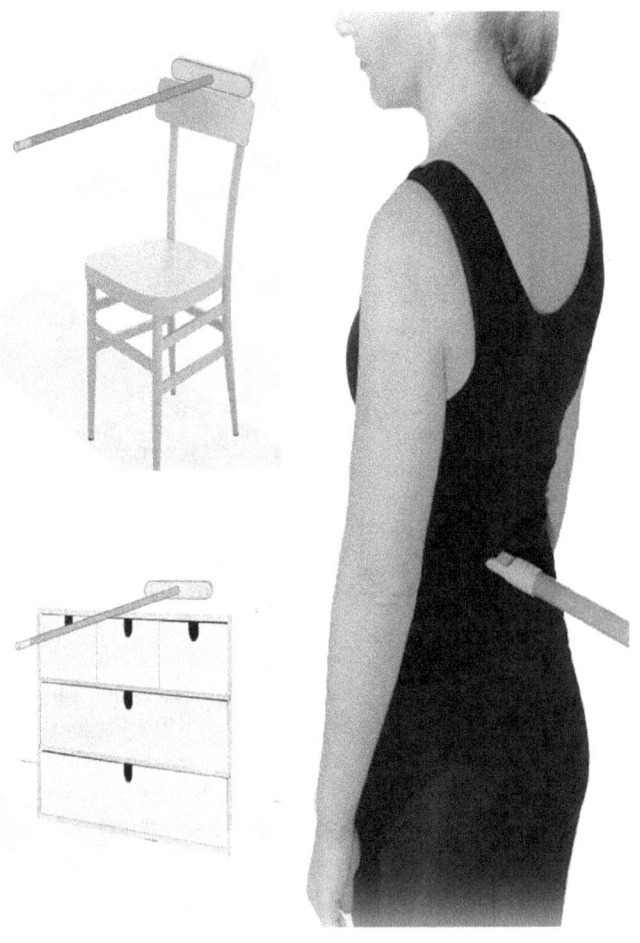

- To treat the pain of the gluteal muscles, it is suitable to use the broom handle or bucket leaned on the corner between the wall and the floor. For

a deeper massaging effect, you can treat painful
points from different angles.

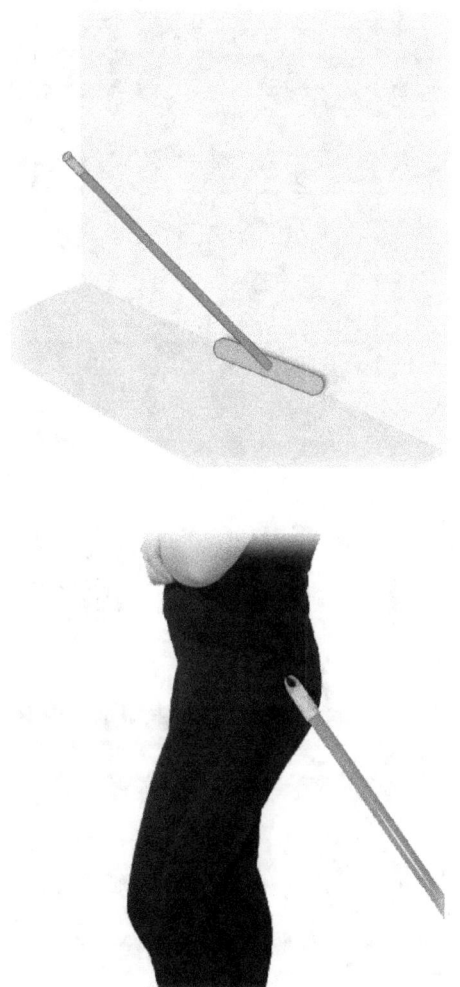

If it is difficult to reach the points on the feet, for this use
a hard round object such as a golf ball, chestnut, round

stone, lid from a shampoo bottle, etc.

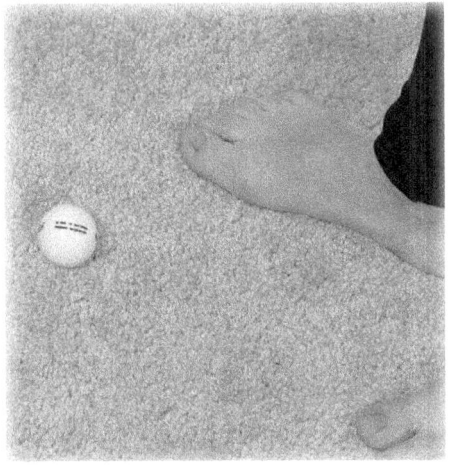

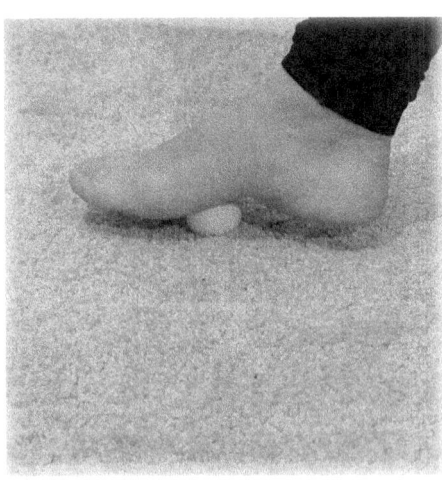

After you have pressed all the points in the painful area, perform the exercises to stretch the muscles of this area.

# CHAPTER 2. STRETCHING THE MUSCLES

## General information

The aim of most of the following exercises is therapeutic stretching of specific muscle groups, supporting blood circulation and the flowing of other body fluids, particularly lymph, eliminating the pain, improving immunity and flexibility. In addition, it is a great way to eliminate mental tension and stress.

### How to stretch muscles properly

1. Doing exercises are to stretch the muscle or group of muscles in that area for which the exercise is designed.

2. Perform all exercises **SLOWLY**!

3. Do not tense up and instead relax to loosen the stretched area, focus on it and close your eyes.

4. Hold the stretch for 15 to 30 seconds until the initial discomfort is reduced. Then, after a period of 5 to 10 seconds, stretch muscles a little more, but do not overstretch. The pain of stretching the muscles must be "good".

5. Perform each stretching exercise two or three times to get a deeper effect. After each exercise, there is reduced pain. Increase muscle tension up to a good feeling and then rest for 15-30 seconds. Next, repeat the stretch if possible with a little more force and with more range.

**Attention**! If you feel a sharp intense pain during an exercise, stop that exercise immediately and consult with a doctor.

## "Magic" cord

For performing a few of the exercises requires a simple tool, nicknamed the *magic cord* by most of my patients.

You need a four meter cord with a diameter of 8-12 mm to make a magic cord.

1. Make a small loop with the length about 15-20 cm folded at one end.

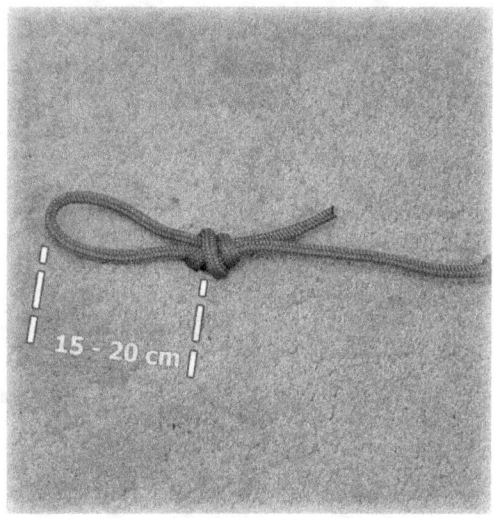

2. Make 4-5 knots under the loop at a distance of 20-25 cm.

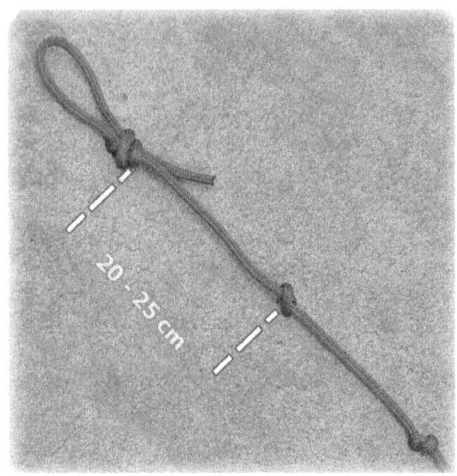

3. Make a large loop at the other end of the cord as follows: bend your leg at the knee, insert your foot over the cord and hold it, and tie a knot over the knee.

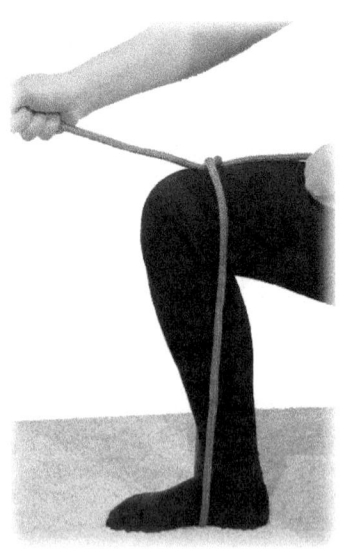

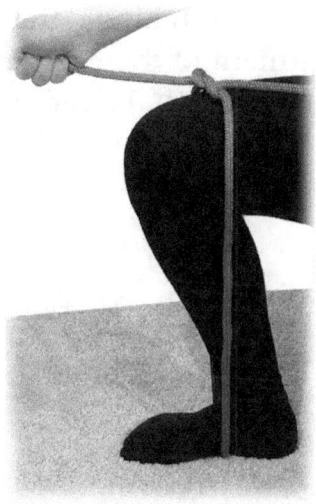

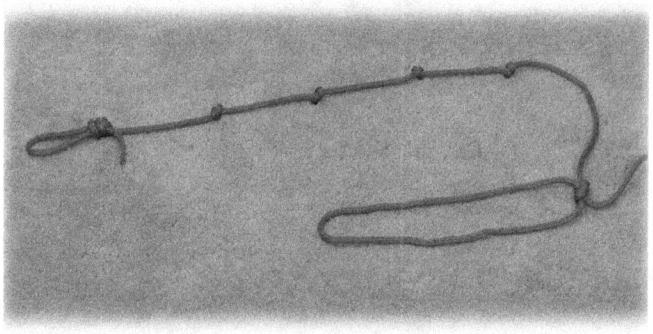

**Attention**! Do not tight the knots immediately and do not dispose of the remains of the cord. Firstly, test an exercise with it. Your physical condition may require a shortening of the cord, lengthening, shifting knots or to separate the large loop from the knots.

# Exercises for stretching, strengthening and treatment of the neck muscles, cervical spine and the thoracic spine

## Exercise 1

The aim of this exercise is to stretch the muscles at the back of the neck and lateral muscles, leading along the thoracic spine.

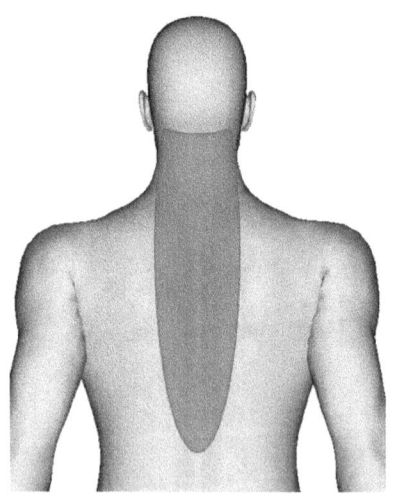

1. *Basic position:* Sit down on chair and keep your back straight. Bend your head forward. Lock your fingers and put your hands to your neck. Hands are relaxed, elbows down.

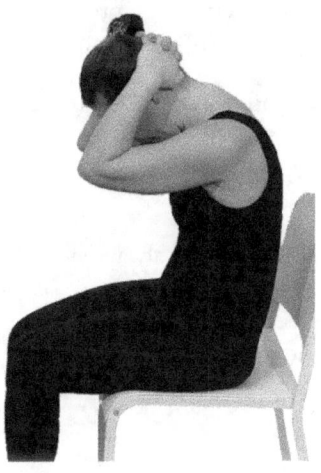

2. Press down on head only by hand force until you feel acceptable pain in the stretched area and relax the muscles of the neck and upper chest. Hold for about 10 to 15 seconds.

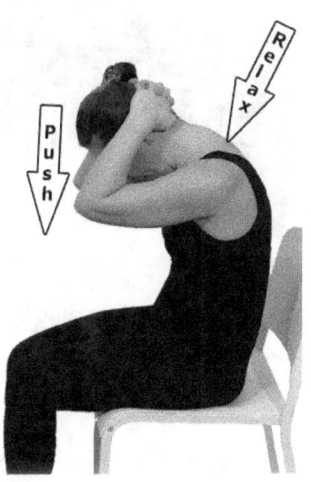

3. After the disappearance of the unpleasant (painful) feeling in the stretched muscles, press your hands to the back of the neck for 10 to 15 seconds.

**Attention**! Neck and back muscles are always **RELAXED** during this exercise!

4. Bend forward slowly, and always stop and relax for a few seconds before the disappearance of the uncomfortable feeling. Thus, you can stretch your back muscles up to the waist.

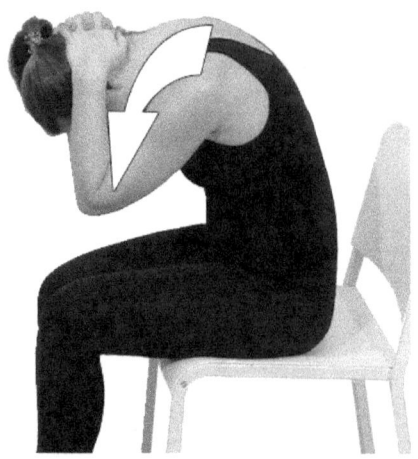

5. Notice: you can exercise in a standing position.

**Exercise 2**

The aim of this exercise is stretching the muscles on the side of the neck

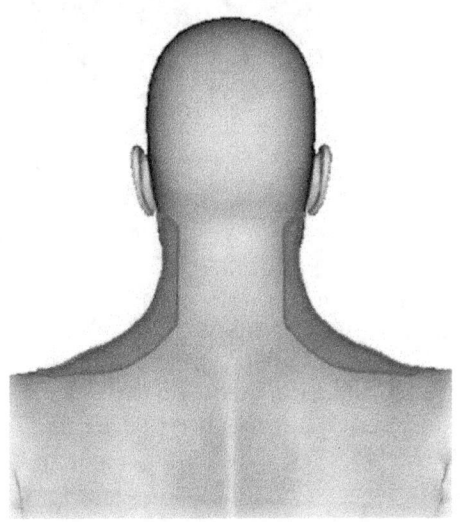

1. *Basic position*: sit down on chair and keep your back straight. Hold the seat of the chair by the hand.

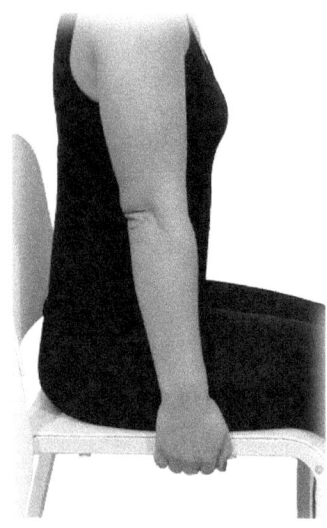

2. Hold a chair, hanging your hands down by your side. Lay your head on the shoulder.

Hold your head with the other hand and pull it toward your shoulder until you feel an acceptable pain in the stretched area. Hold such position for about 10 to 15 seconds.

**Attention**! The stretched area is **RELAXED**!

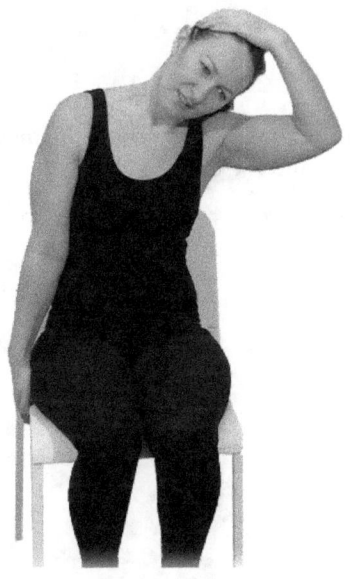

3. Change your hands and stretch on other side.

4. Repeat the exercise two to three times on each side.

**Exercise 3**

The aim of this exercise is stretching the muscles on the lower-neck side and the cervical spine

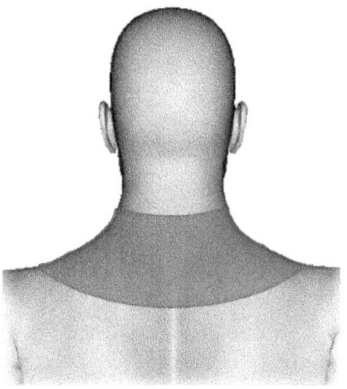

1. *Basic position:* sit down on a chair and keep your back straight. Hold the seat of the chair by the hands, and a little to the back of you.

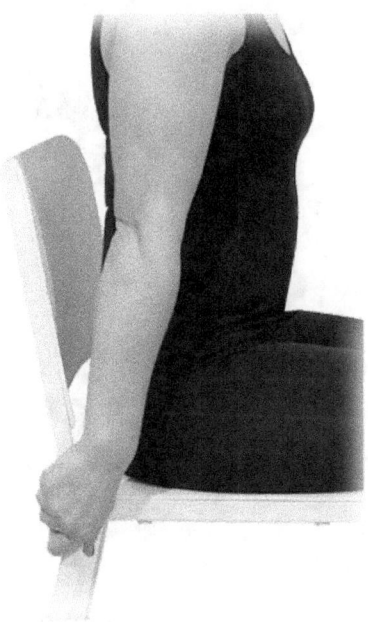

2. Hold the chair and lean your head forward and to a shoulder.

Hold your head with the other hand and pull it forward and to your shoulder until you feel an acceptable pain in the stretched area. Stay in such position for about 10 to 15 seconds.

**Attention**! The stretched area is **RELAXED**!

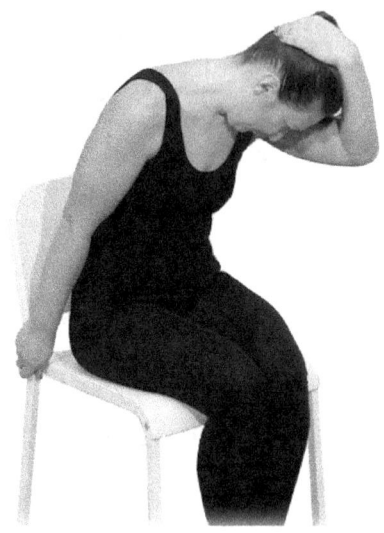

3. Change your hands and stretch the other side.


4. Repeat the exercise two to three times on each side.

**Exercise 4**

The aim of this exercise is stretching the muscles on the upper neck

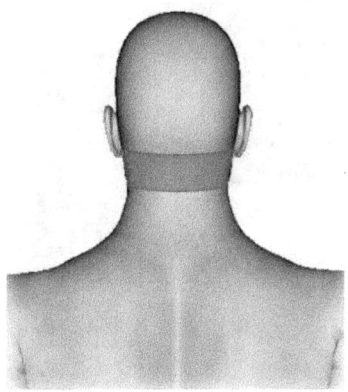

1. *Basic position*: sit down on a chair and keep your back straight. Hold the seat of the chair by the hand, and a little forward.

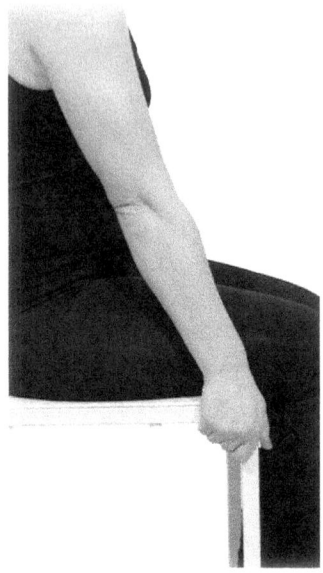

2. Hold the chair and lean your head back and to a shoulder.

Hold your head with the other hand and pull it back and to your shoulder until you feel an acceptable amount of pain in the stretched area. Hold on to such position for about 10 to 15 seconds.

**Attention**! The stretched area is **RELAXED**!

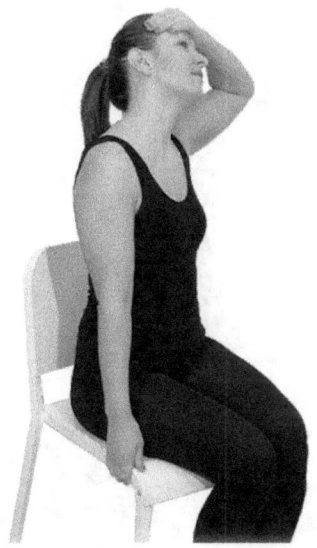

3. Change your hands and stretch on other side.


4. Repeat the exercise three to five times on each side.

**Exercise 5**

The aim of this exercise is stretching the muscles on the central side of the neck.

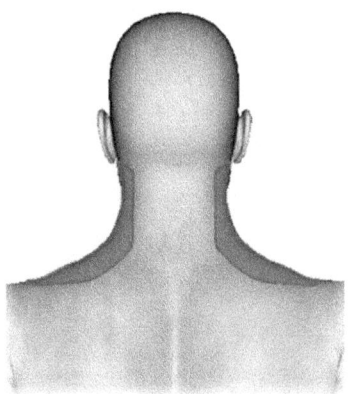

1. *Basic position*: sit down on a chair and keep your back straight. Put your hands down and keep your head in a vertical position.

2. Lean your ear to your shoulder.

3. Pull your muscles of second ear up, like when someone pulls up behind your ear. Shoulders must remain in the same level.

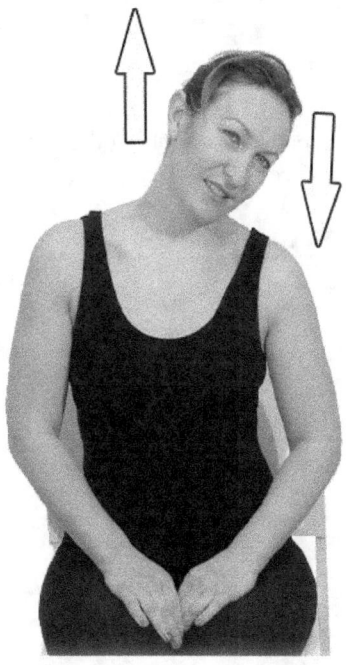

4. Change your hands and stretch on other side.


5. Repeat the exercise three to five times on each side.

**Exercise 6**

The aim of this exercise is stretching the muscles of the lower-neck and the cervical spine.

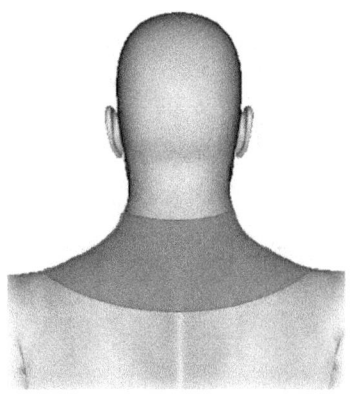

1. *Basic position*: sit down on a chair and keep your back straight with your hands down.

2. Lean your head forward at maximum and pull your ear down to your shoulder.

3. Pull your muscles of the other ear forward, like when someone pulls up behind your ear. Shoulders must remain in the same level.

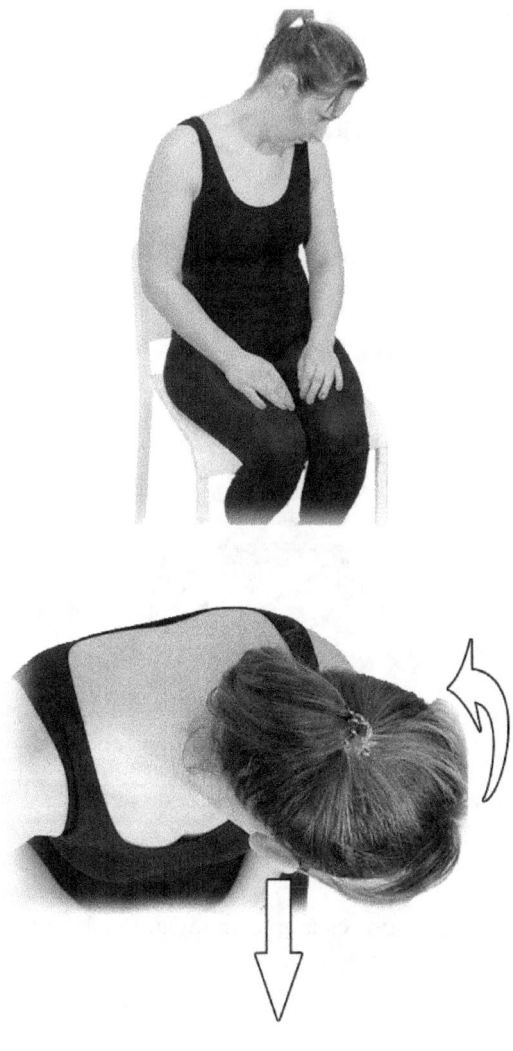

4. Change your hands and stretch on other side.


5. Repeat the exercise three to five times on each side.

**Exercise 7**

The aim of this exercise is stretching the muscles of the upper neck.

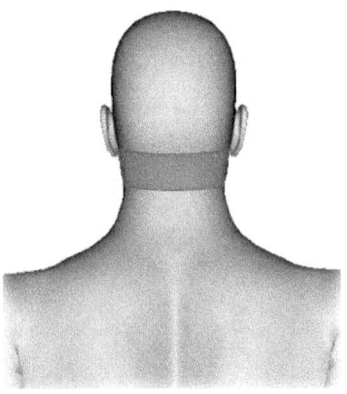

1. *Basic position:* sit down on chair and keep your back straight with your hands down.

2. Lean your head back at maximum and pull your ear down to your shoulder.

3. Pull your muscles of second ear back, like when someone pulls up behind your ear. Shoulders must remain in the same level.

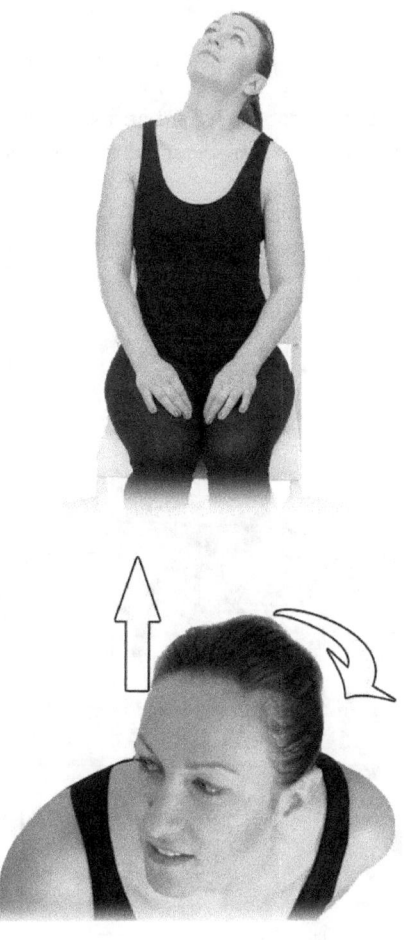

4. Change your hands and stretch on other side.

5. Repeat the exercise three to five times on each side.

**Exercise 8**

The aim of this exercise is to treat and support the muscles on the upper part of the thoracic spine (between the shoulder blades).

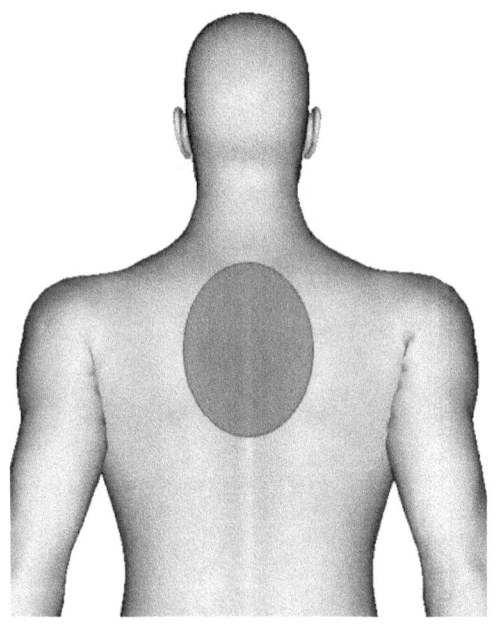

1. *Basic position*: sit down on a chair and keep your back straight. Lean your head forward to maximum. Lock your hands and put it on the scruff of the neck with the elbows down.

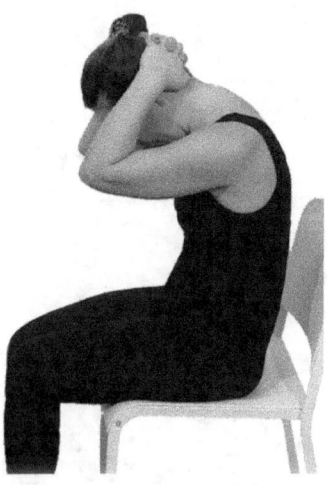

2. Press your head by the hands and oppose the raise of your head using both the hands.

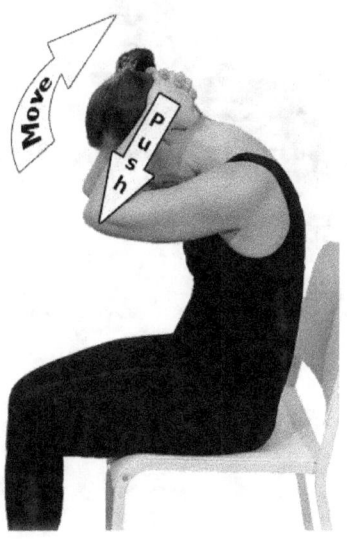

3. When your head is in normal position, put your elbows out to the sides to the max.

**Attention**! Move your head from the beginning to the end without stopping. The pressure of your hands should be consistent.

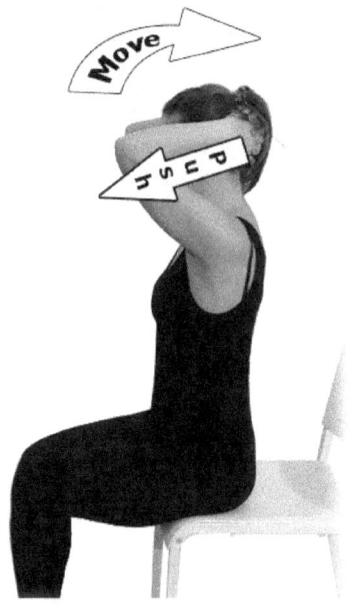

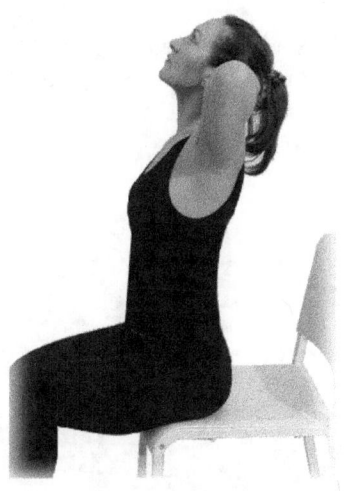

4. Repeat the exercise two to three times.

**Exercise 9**

The aim of this exercise is stretching of the neck muscles, cervical spine and upper part of the spine in the back.

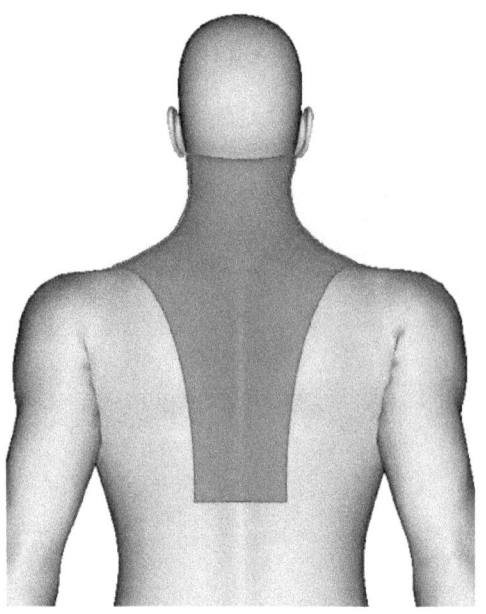

1. *Basic position*: sit down on a chair and keep your back straight. Lean your head forward at maximum.

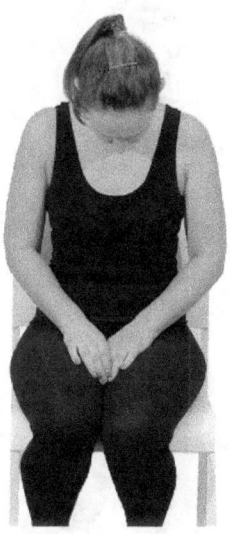

2. Stretch your muscles slowly and stop at the points of tension, move your head around from the shoulder, then back, then on the other shoulder and to the front.

Alex Taurus

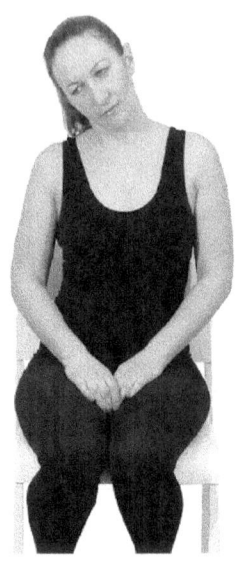

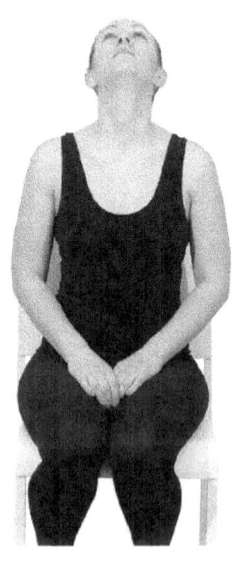

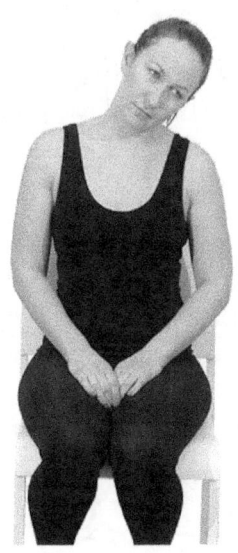

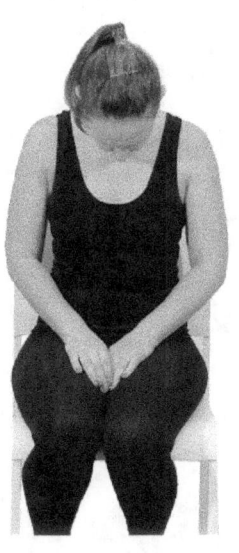

3. Repeat the same movement to the other side.

4. Repeat the exercise two to three times.

# Exercises for stretching, strengthening and treatment of muscles of the shoulder joint, chest muscles and muscles of the hand

## Exercise 1

The aim of this exercise is stretching the chest muscles, shoulder muscles, biceps and muscles of the forearm.

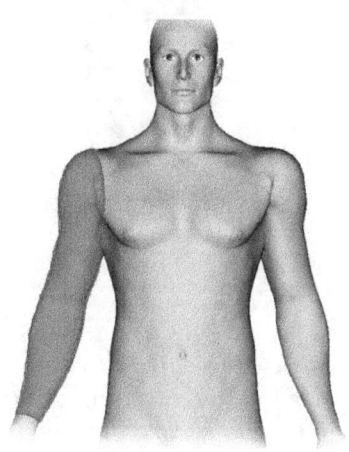

1. *Basic position*: stand up at a half step away from the wall. Raise your hand about 45° and lean your hands with fingers up against the wall.

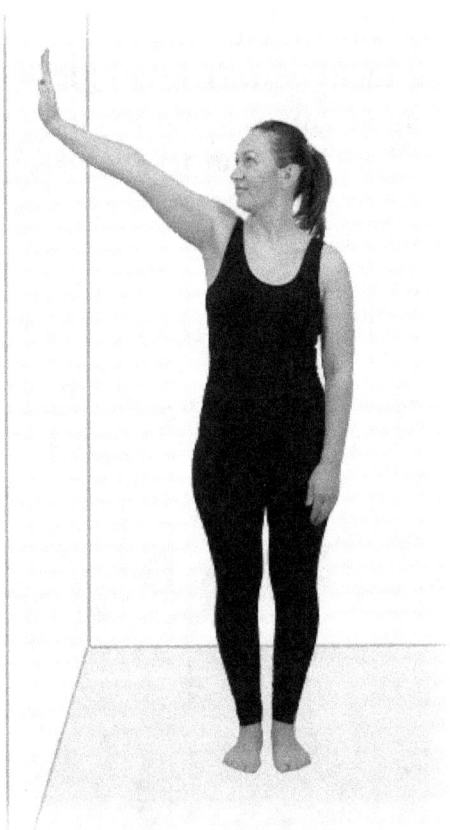

2. Hold your hand in the same place and rotate around at vertical axis slowly away from the raised arm with the other hand moving forward until you feel an acceptable level of pain in the stretched area. Hold on for 10 to 15 seconds.

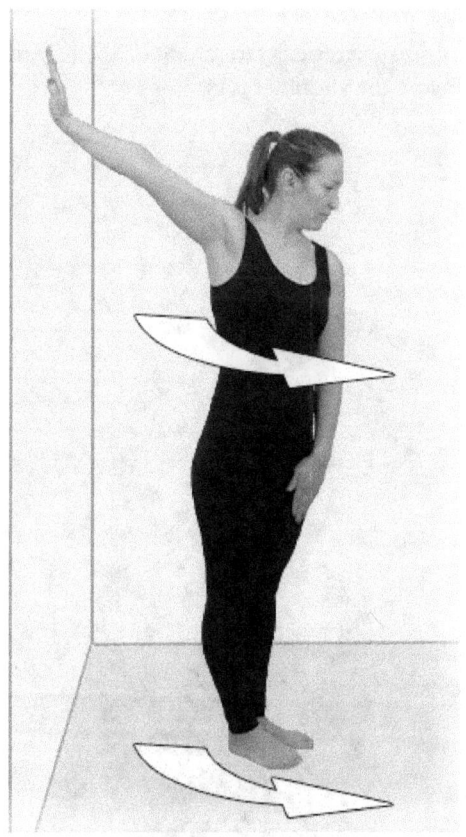

3. Change your hands and stretch the other side.

4. Repeat the exercise two to three times on each side.

## Exercise 2

The aim of this exercise is stretching of the triceps and muscles below the shoulder joint.

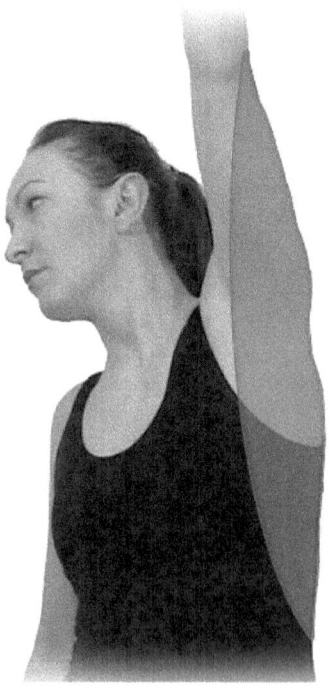

1. *Basic position*: Stand in the doorway, lift the left hand and grab the top edge of the frame.
If, because of small stature, you cannot get to the top of the doorway, use something with a lower height for this exercise, such as the lower part of a flight of stairs or a handrail.

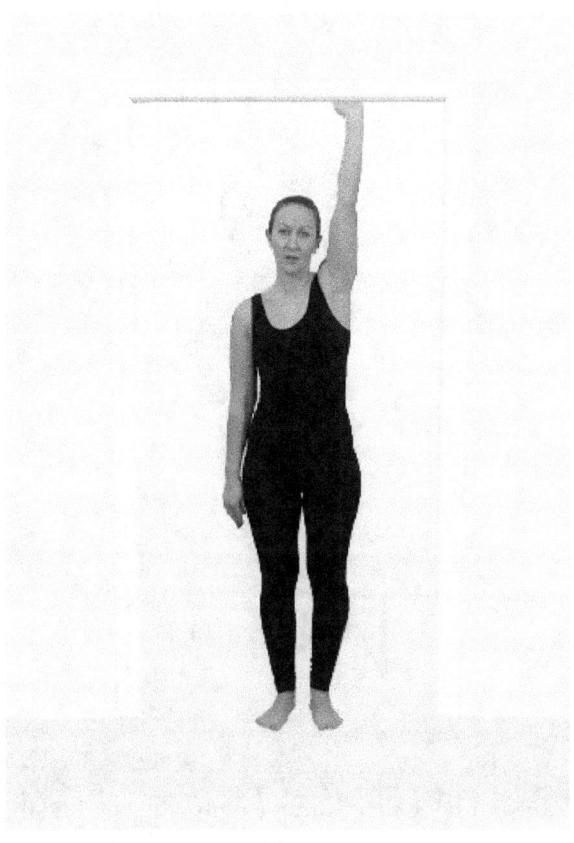

2. Take the right foot one step forward and flex the body forward.

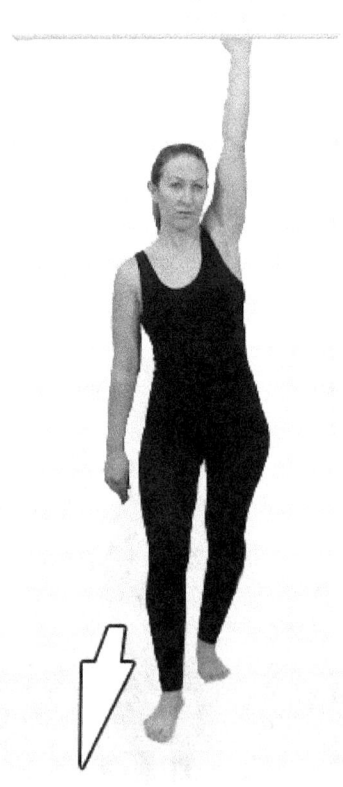

3. Turn your body slightly to the right until you find the muscles that are most contracted (those places you feel muscle discomfort). Keep muscles tensed for 10 to 15 seconds.

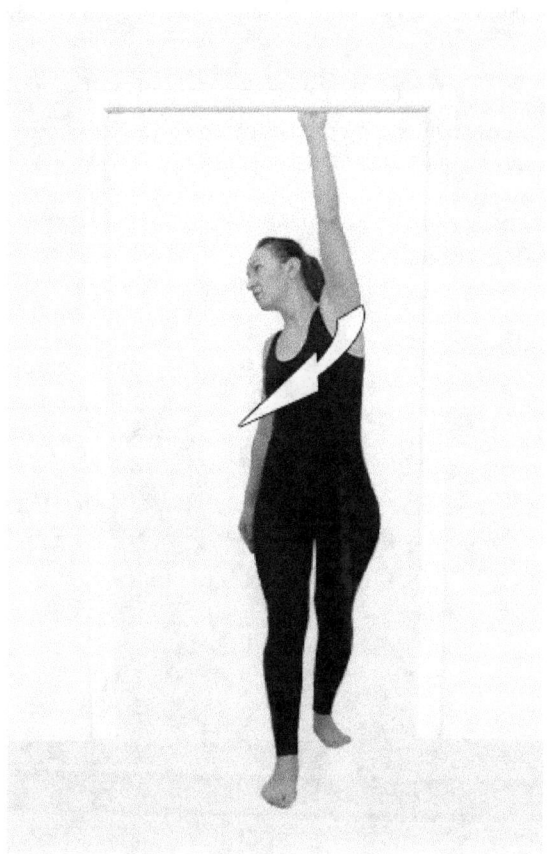

4. Change your hands and stretch the other side.

5. Repeat the exercise two to three times on each side.

**Exercise 3**

The aim of this exercise is stretching of the front part of the shoulder joint.

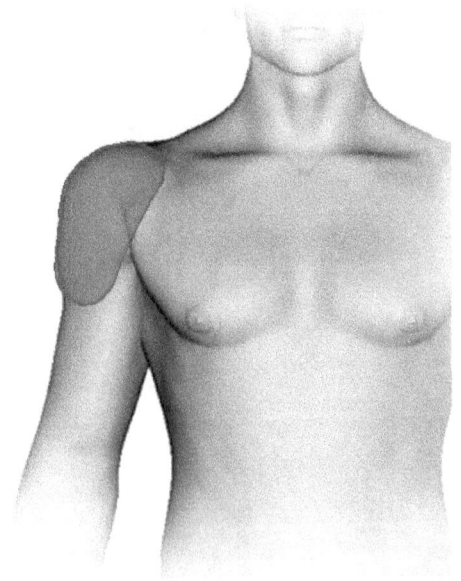

This exercise requires a cylindrical item with a diameter of 7 to 10 cm and a towel. For instance, use plastic bottles of water, rolled-up towel or blanket, etc.

1. *Basic position*: put your right hand behind your back and insert a cylinder between the wrist and back.

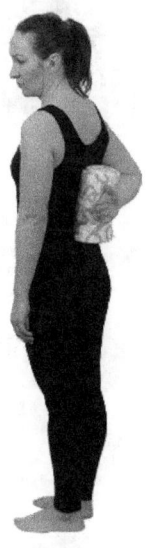

2. Sling a towel over your left shoulder hold both ends of the towel.

3. Pull up your right arm with a towel by your left hand until you feel an acceptable pain in the stretched area. Pull down the towel by your left hand to fix this position.

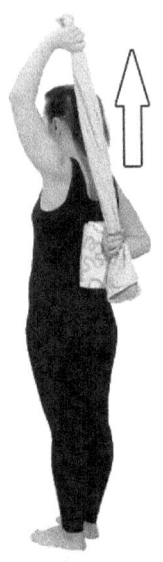

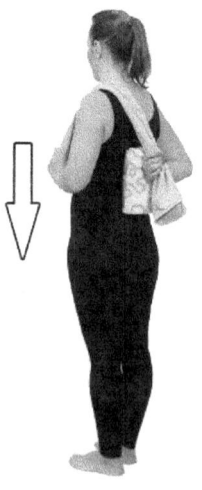

4. Pull the towel down by your right hand and hold for 8 to 10 seconds.

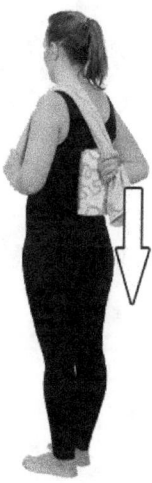

5. Then, loosen a little and pull up the towel with your right hand with your left hand. Remain in this position and pull the towel down again for 8 to 10 seconds. Relax.

6. Repeat steps three and four for, two to five times for the pain in the shoulder, but do not overdo it.

7. Change your hands and perform the same exercise with your other hand.

**Exercise 4**

The aim of this exercise is stretching of the muscles of the upper part of the forearm.

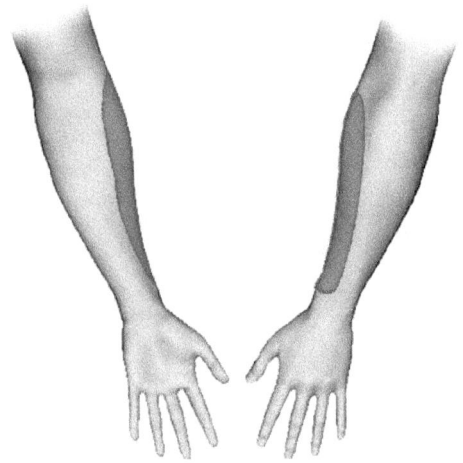

1. *Basic position*: stand up near the table. Lean the outer edge of your palm side on the table, palm facing outward. Pull the elbow with the other hand and straighten hand.

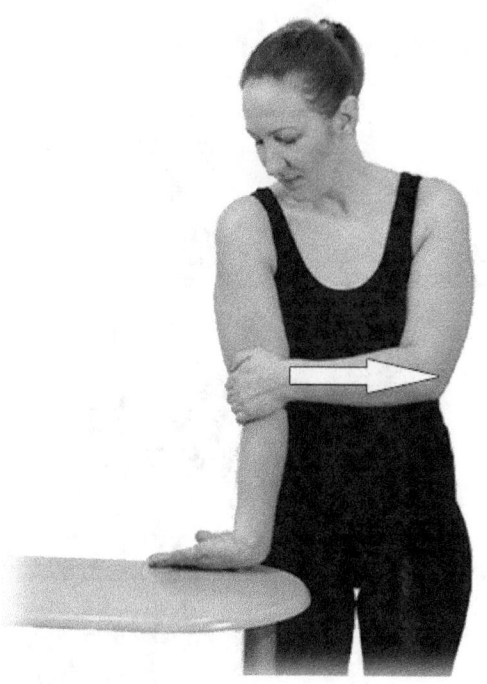

2. Constantly pull the elbow, leave your palm in the same place, and bow toward with your body slowly in the direction of your fingers until you feel an acceptable level of pain in the stretched area. Hold on for 10 to 15 seconds.

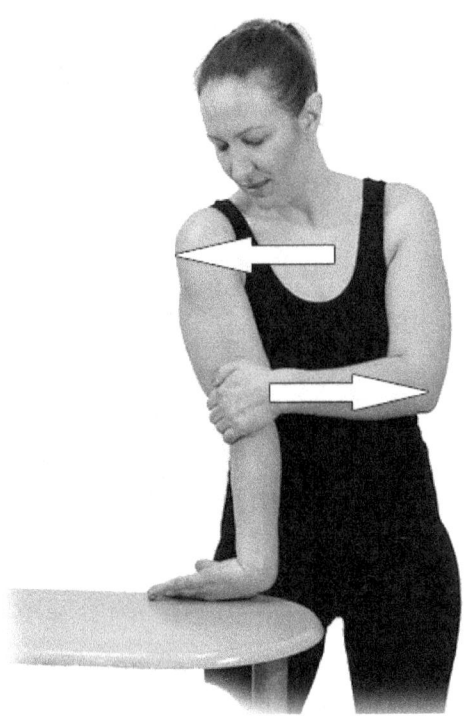

3. Change your hands and stretch your other hand.

4. Repeat the exercise two to three times with each hand.

**Exercise 5**

The aim of this exercise is stretching of the group of the muscles of the central part of the forearm.

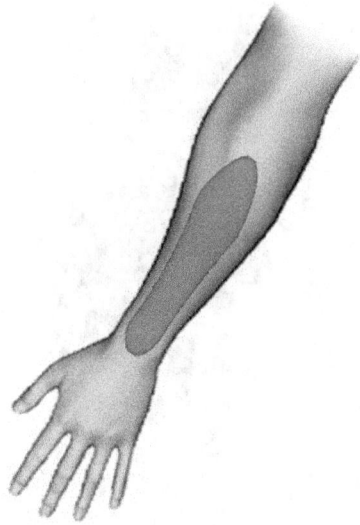

1. *Basic position*: stand up near the table. Lean the outer side of your palm on the table, palm facing to you. Pull the elbow with the other hand and straighten hand.

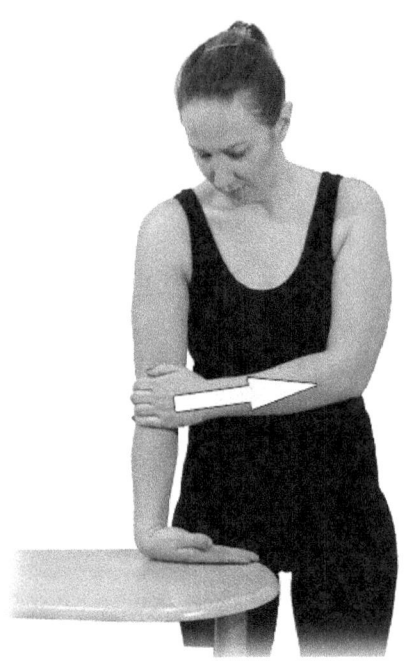

2. Constantly pull the elbow, leave your palm in the same place, and lean your body slowly in the direction of your fingers until you feel an acceptable level of pain in the stretched area. Hold for 10 to 15 seconds.

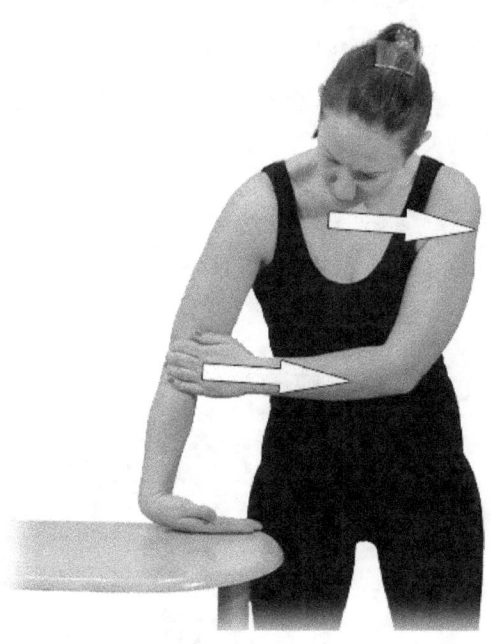

3. Change your hands and stretch your other hand.

4. Repeat the exercise two to three times with each hand.

**Exercise 6**

The aim of this exercise is stretching of the group of muscles of the forearm.

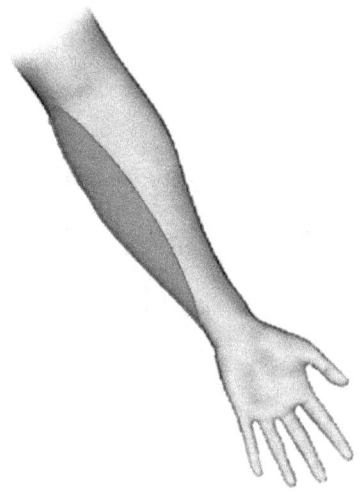

1. *Basic position*: sit down at the table. Lean the bent elbow of your hand on the table, palm facing upwards, fingers outward.

2. Hold your fingers by the second hand and press down until you feel an acceptable level of pain in the stretched area. Hold for 10 to 15 seconds.

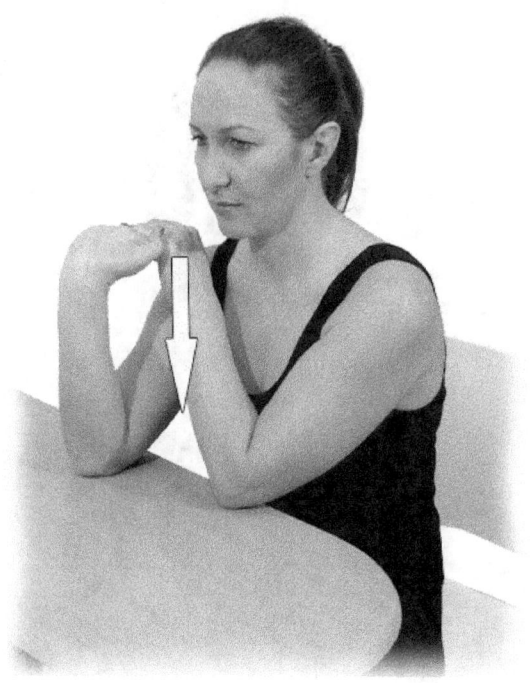

3. It is more effective when you press on the arm with your chin.

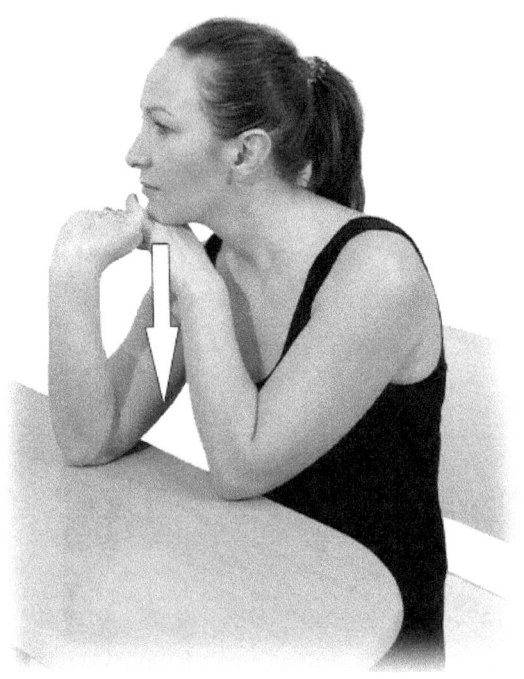

4. Change your hands and stretch your other hand.

5. Repeat the exercise two to three times with each hand.

# Exercises for stretching, treatment and strengthening the muscles of the lower half of the body. Lumbar spine, buttocks and legs.

**Exercise 1**

The aim of this exercise is stretching of the muscles of the back of the thigh and shin.

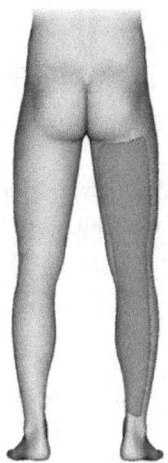

1. *Basic position*: sit down on the floor, put your heel into a small loop of the magic cord, put the cord between the first and second toe of the foot.

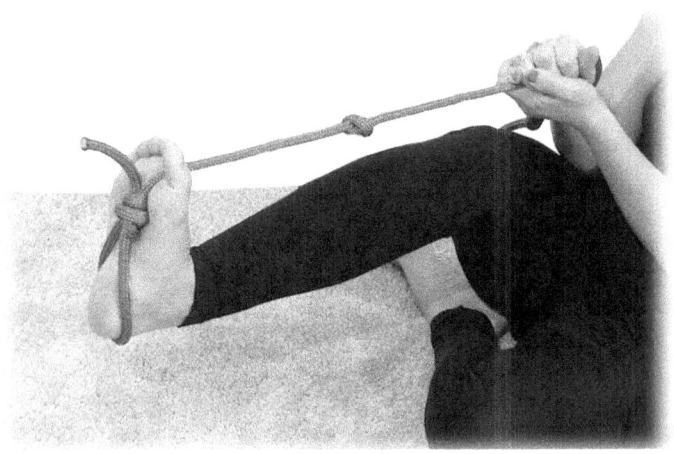

2. Lie on your back, hold the cord in your hand.

3. Raise the stretched leg up to maximum.

4. Pull the cord towards you with one hand, and extend your leg away until you feel an acceptable level of pain in the stretched area.

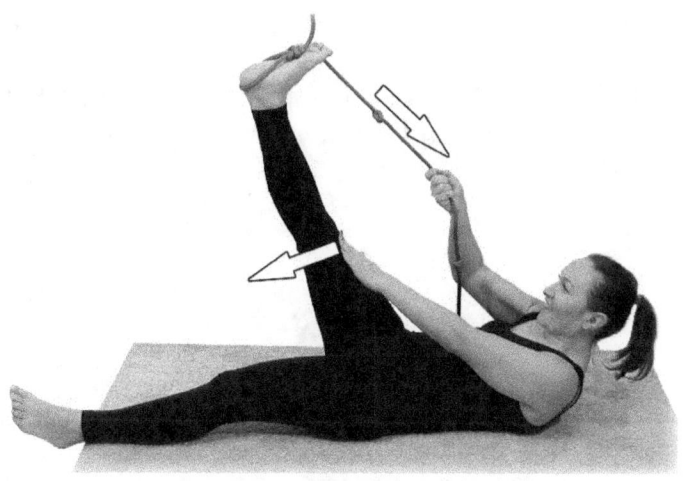

5. Try to relax the stretched muscles and hold on for 15 to 30 seconds. Then, return your foot down to the ground and relax for 10 to 15 seconds. Repeat this exercise two to three times.

6. Change legs and repeat the exercise from the beginning.

If it is difficult for you to press your leg with your hands because of height of the raised leg, pull the cord with both hands and try to keep the leg straight (do not bend your knee).

## Exercise 2

The aim of this exercise is for stretching of the lateral thigh muscles, gluteal muscles and the lower part of the lumbar spine.

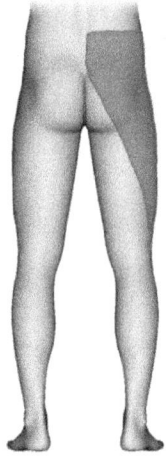

**Option 1**

1. *Basic position*: lie flat on the floor face up, shoulder blade pushing upward.

2. Lift the bent leg at the knee and place it over the other leg until the foot reaches the floor, the heel closest to the knee where heel of one foot and the opposite knee creates

a "lock".

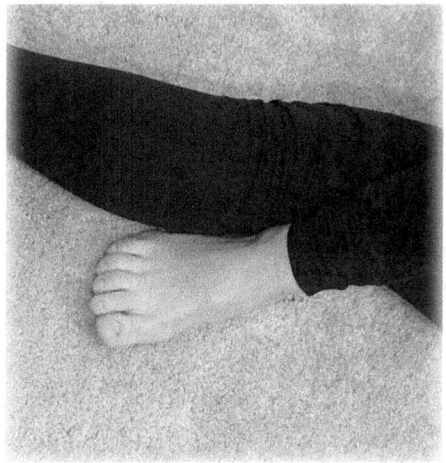

3. Hold your knee in your hand and stretch it to the floor and to yourself until you feel an acceptable level of pain in the stretched area.

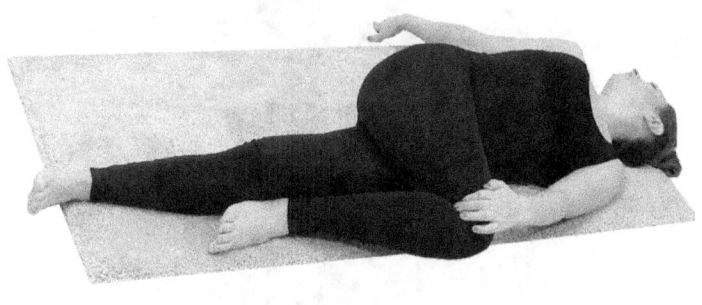

4. Try to relax the stretched muscles, hold on for 15 to 30

seconds. Then, return your foot down to the floor, relax for 10 to 15 seconds and repeat the exercise two to three times.

5. Replace the leg with the other leg and repeat the exercise from the beginning.

If you cannot reach the knee or if you don't have enough strength to press, use a larger loop of the magic cord.

## Option 2

1. *Basic position*: sit down on the floor, put your knee and heel into a large loop of the magic cord. Lie down on the floor with your shoulder blade pressing upwards.

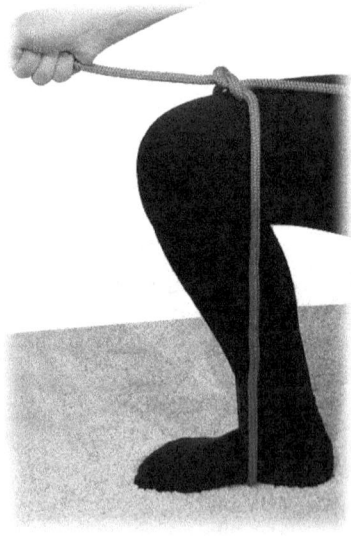

2. Lift the bent leg at the knee and place it over the other leg until the foot reaches the floor, the heel closest to the knee where heel of one foot and the opposite knee creates a "lock".

3. Hold the loop on your knee by the hand and stretch it to the floor and to yourself until you feel an acceptable pain in the stretched area.

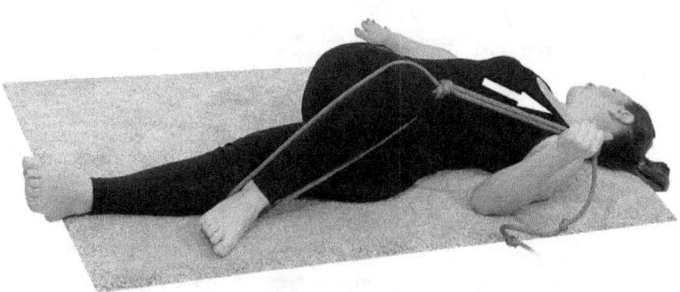

4. Try to relax the stretched muscles, hold for 15 to 30 seconds. Then, return your foot down to the floor, relax for 10 to 15 seconds and repeat the exercise two to three times.

5. Replace the leg with the other one and repeat the exercise from the beginning.

**Attention**! If you feel a sharp pain in the groin area, discontinue the exercise immediately and consult with a doctor (for examination of the hip joint).

**Exercise 3**

The aim of this exercise is stretching of the lateral and back thigh muscles, shins, gluteal muscles and the muscles of the lumbar spine.

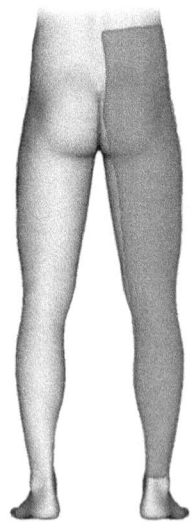

1. *Basic position*: sit down on the floor, put your heel into a little loop of the magic cord, and put the cord between the first and second toes. Lie down on your back and stretch cord with your hand with your shoulder blade pressing to the floor.

2. Lift the stretched leg and put it over the other leg.

3. Try to hold your foot at the lowest position as far as possible (as close to the floor), pull the cord towards yourself until you feel an acceptable level pain in the stretched area.

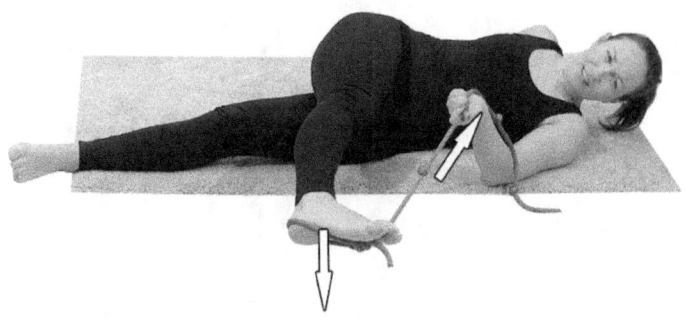

4. Try to relax the stretched muscles, and hold for 15 to 30 seconds. Then, return your foot down, relax for 10 to 15 seconds and repeat the exercise two to three times.

5. Replace the leg with the other one and repeat the exercise from the beginning.

**Attention**! If you feel a sharp pain in the groin area, discontinue the exercise immediately and consult with a doctor (for examination of the hip joint).

If your condition does not allow you put one leg over the other too far, do it slowly and increase the angle gradually.

**Exercise 4**

The aim of this exercise is stretching of the internal thigh muscles.

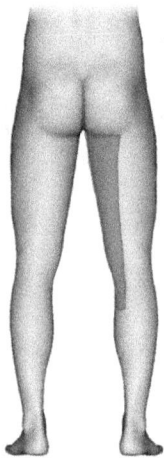

1. *Basic position*: sit down on the floor, put your heel into a little loop of the magic cord, and put the cord between the first and second toes. Lie down on your back and stretch cord into your hands with your shoulder blade pressing to the floor.

2. Lift and stretch a leg at about 45° and put it to the side.

3. Try to turn the toes of your foot to the floor, and pull the cord until you feel an acceptable level of pain in the stretched area.

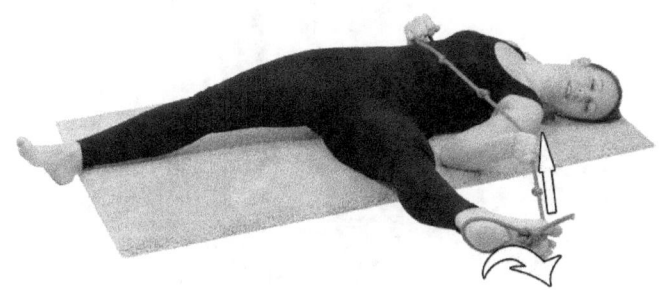

4. Try to relax the stretched muscles, hold on for 15 to 30 seconds. Then, return your foot down to the floor, relax for 10 to 15 seconds and repeat the exercise two to three times.

5. Replace the leg with the other one and repeat the exercise from the beginning.

**Exercise 5**

The aim of this exercise is stretching of the front thigh muscles.

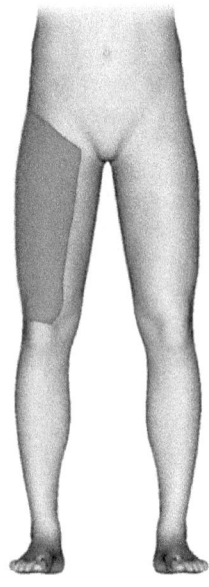

## Option 1

1. 1. *Basic position*: kneel down on your knees and align your feet on the floor.

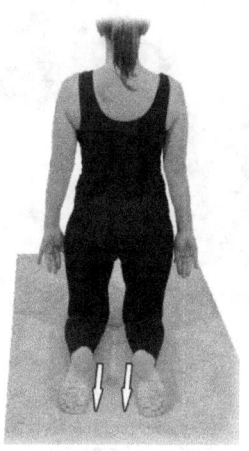

2. Curve your body backwards and lean your hands behind against the floor, shifting your weight on your hands.

3. Flex your hands gradually until you feel an acceptable level of pain in the stretched area.

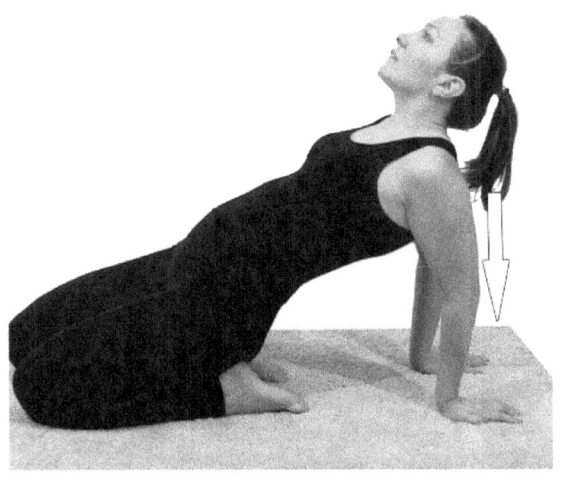

4. Try to relax the stretched muscles, hold on for 15 to 30 seconds. Then, straighten your hands and relax for 10 to 15 seconds. Repeat the exercise two to three times.

If you cannot align your feet on the floor, flex your body back or lean your body on your hands, use the second option for this exercise.

## Option 2

1. *Basic position:* sit down on the floor and put your foot into a little loop of the magic cord.

2. Lie down on your stomach. Now bend your leg at the knees and pull the cord with your hand.

3. Stretch the cord forward until you feel an acceptable level of pain in the stretched area.

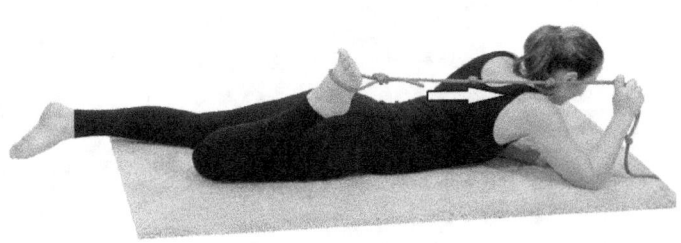

4. Try to relax the stretched muscles, hold for 15 to 30 seconds. Then, return your foot down on the floor and relax for 10 to 15 seconds. Repeat the exercise for two to three times.

5. Replace the leg with the other one and repeat the exercise from the beginning.

For a deeper effect of this exercise, insert anything under your knee, for example, a pillow from the couch, pillow or a rolled blanket, etc., if necessary.

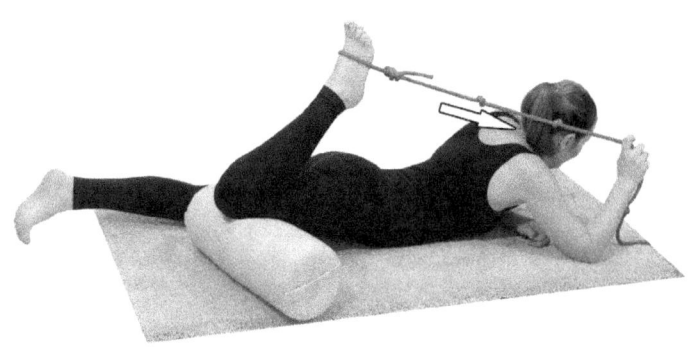

**Exercise 6**

The aim of this exercise is treatment and strengthening of the outer thigh muscles, improving blood circulation in the pelvic organs.

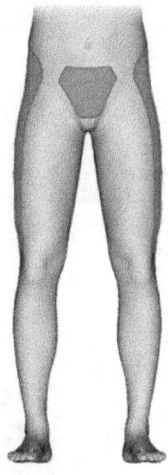

1. *Basic position*: Lie down on your back. Put your legs into a large loop of the magic cord, above the knees. Bend your knees and put your feet on the floor at 25 to 30 cm apart.

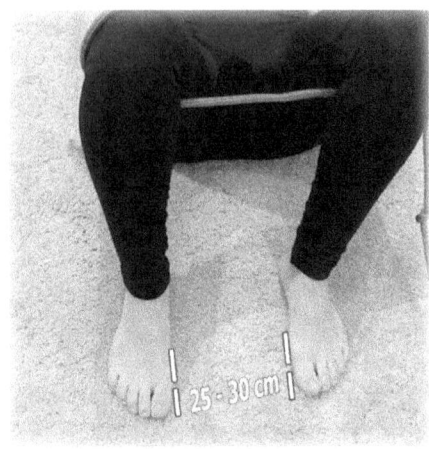

2. Spread your knees out to the sides while the loop is hard stretched, hold on for 10 to 15 seconds.

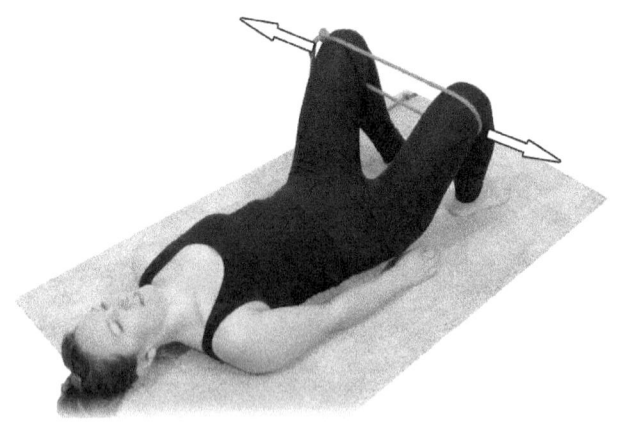

3. Relax for 10 to 15 seconds and repeat the exercise two to three times.

**Exercise 7**

The aim of this exercise is treatment and strengthening of the inner thigh muscles and to improve blood circulation in the pelvic organs.

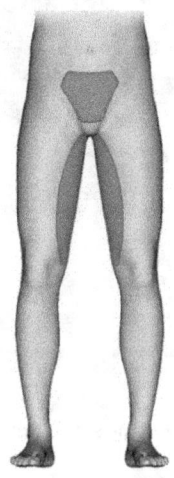

You need a ball (football, volleyball and basketball) to perform this exercise. If you do not have ball, use a pillow from the couch or rolled pillow or blanket, etc.

1. *Basic position:* Lie down on your back. Bend your knees and put your feet on the floor at 25 to 30 cm apart. Press the ball between your knees.

2. Press the ball between knees firmly and hold for 10 to 15 seconds.

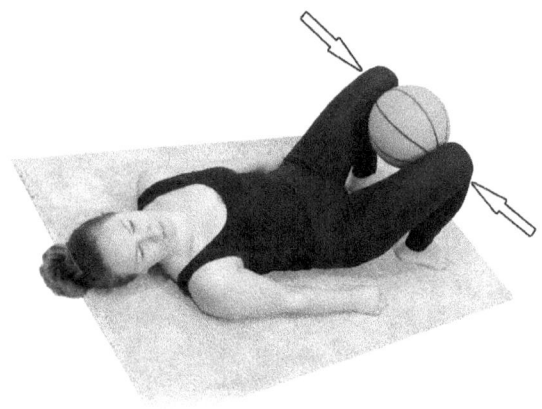

3. Relax for 10 to 15 seconds and repeat the exercise two to three times.